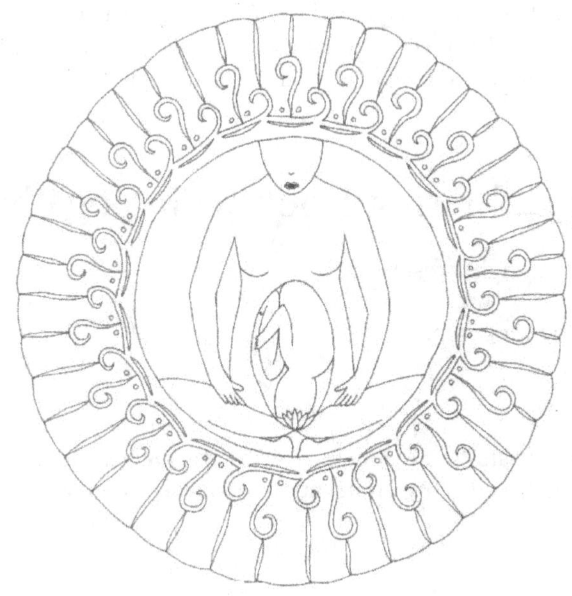

The Pregnancy and Birth Colouring Book
with Yoga Nidra

A colouring book with positive words and guided relaxations to support and enhance your pregnancy, birth and postnatal journey.

Tessa Venuti Sanderson, PhD

Castenetto & Co.

Dedication

Thank you to my mother for birthing me without the benefit of knowing any of this, to Uma Dinsmore-Tuli and Nirlipta Tuli for their inspiration, and to all of the women who have attended my classes and workshops over the years. I dedicate this book to my daughters and my sister – may you be as blessed as I have been.

The Pregnancy and Birth Colouring Book with Yoga Nidra

Second paperback edition 2019 in the United Kingdom.

ISBN 9781687133885

Published by Castenetto & Co.
For more copies of this book, please email: hello@tessayoga.co.uk or visit www.tessayoga.co.uk

Printed by KDP.

Although every precaution has been taken in the preparation of this book, the publisher and author assume no responsibility for errors or omissions. Neither is any liability assumed for damages resulting from the use of this information contained herein.

Contents page

Introduction

My aim for this colouring book is to provide an emotional space for you to reflect on your pregnancy, birth and postnatal journey. By colouring in these images of pregnancy and birth, you can access the intuitive part of your mind and connect with your innermost feelings.

We are bombarded by information about pregnancy and birth in the modern world. By connecting with your creative nature through colouring, and while considering the positive words alongside the pictures, you can focus on creating a calm confidence about your ability to birth your baby naturally.

While colouring the mandalas and listening to the Yoga Nidra (relaxation) tracks, you are using your senses of sight, touch and hearing. Smelling relaxing essential oils and tasting nourishing foods at the same time will give you a complete sensory experience!

The mandalas

The pictures in the book are enclosed within mandalas. A mandala is a sacred circle. A circle represents a safe container, so that the different images of pregnancy and birth are at the same time protected and made special. Birth is a rite of passage for women; a transition to becoming a different person, and therefore sacred in your life journey.

The mandalas are hand drawn and therefore not perfect, just as many births do not proceed 'perfectly' or exactly how we imagined they would be. A famous Persian proverb states: "The Persian carpet is perfectly imperfect, and precisely imprecise". This phrase comes from their belief that only God can create perfection.

I have not drawn the women's faces in detail, so that you can better visualise yourself in each of the positions.

I believe that it is wise to gather many tools together to support you during birth (whether it be breathing techniques, yoga postures, hypnobirthing, and so on) and perhaps to write down your birth preferences. However, at some point it is important to let go of your expectations as a precursor to letting go physically of the baby you have carried within, and to keep on letting go of the child as s/he becomes more independent.

Be creative

I have included space for you to create a mandala of your own. You might draw an image in the centre or use magazine pictures to make a collage, then doodle around the circle to create the mandala. You can add your own words: perhaps you could write an affirmation to address a particular anxiety. Write it in the present tense (as if it were already true) and using positive language. The shorter it is, the better. For example, "I trust my body to birth my baby", rather than "I do not worry about my birth and will not listen to negative stories"! Every time that you hear yourself or someone say something negative about birth, repeat your affirmation to provide a positive feedback loop. Ideas for affirmations or intentions around your pregnancy and birth can be found in this book, including the Yoga Nidra (relaxation) scripts at the back of the book.

You can photocopy the pages from the book for your own use, so that you can colour the mandalas in multiple times or colour them with your toddler to explain what will happen when the new baby is coming. If you are using the mandalas for a birth art session or antenatal classes, please use up to two of the images to share with others stating their source, but no more at any one time. It is ideal to put the coloured mandalas in a place that you will frequently see them, to reinforce their positive messages. For example, you could stick them to the wall where you will see them when you first wake up.

Yoga Nidra for pregnancy – "Nidrabirthing"

In the scripts at the back of the book, I guide you through a technique called Yoga Nidra. The effect of this relaxing, meditative process is to allow your physical body to totally rest, while your mind is invited to settle into theta brain waves. Both scripts act as guided relaxations to support your pregnancy, particularly in the last trimester.

I have specially constructed two scripts: the first, shorter one is about birth being a natural process and is ideal to listen to with your partner. The second, slightly longer one is for you, the pregnant woman. The latter guides you in using many of the book's images such as flowers blooming, waves and mountains, in order to support you through different stages of your birthing journey.

You can listen to these guided relaxations, by downloading the audio tracks at www.tessayoga.co.uk/colouringbookdownloads. Alternatively, you or someone whose voice you enjoy, can read the scripts and record it for yourself.

I recommend listening to the Yoga Nidra before colouring in for maximum benefit, if you have access to recordings and the time to lie down. This will support the reflective process as you use the book; see how you react to the different images and accompanying words. However, you can also have the tracks playing as you colour in and during the birthing journey itself.

For instructions on how to lie for Yoga Nidra when pregnant, and instructions for maximising its benefit, please turn to the end of the book.

What I have written is not meant to be prescriptive, but are suggestions for a positive pregnancy and birthing journey. It is very beneficial to attend a local pregnancy yoga class with a qualified teacher. The positions are intended for a woman with a normal, healthy pregnancy. Please consult your medical practitioner if you are unsure whether anything in the book is unsuitable in your particular circumstances.

Finally, best wishes for your pregnancy, birth and transition into becoming a mother (again).

I hope that this resource will support you in your journey.

Tessa

Om namaha shivaya

With great respect and love, I honour my heart, my inner teacher.

Tessa is the mother of two daughters, both born in water, one at home. She is a a yoga teacher, specialising in Pregnancy, Mother & Baby and Well Woman Yoga: www.tessayoga.co.uk. She is also a Menstrual Educator, teaching girls and women about menstrual cycle awareness: www.cyclicalwisdom.com. She has a PhD in Medical Sociology and has published over 20 academic publications.

Breathing and Blooming

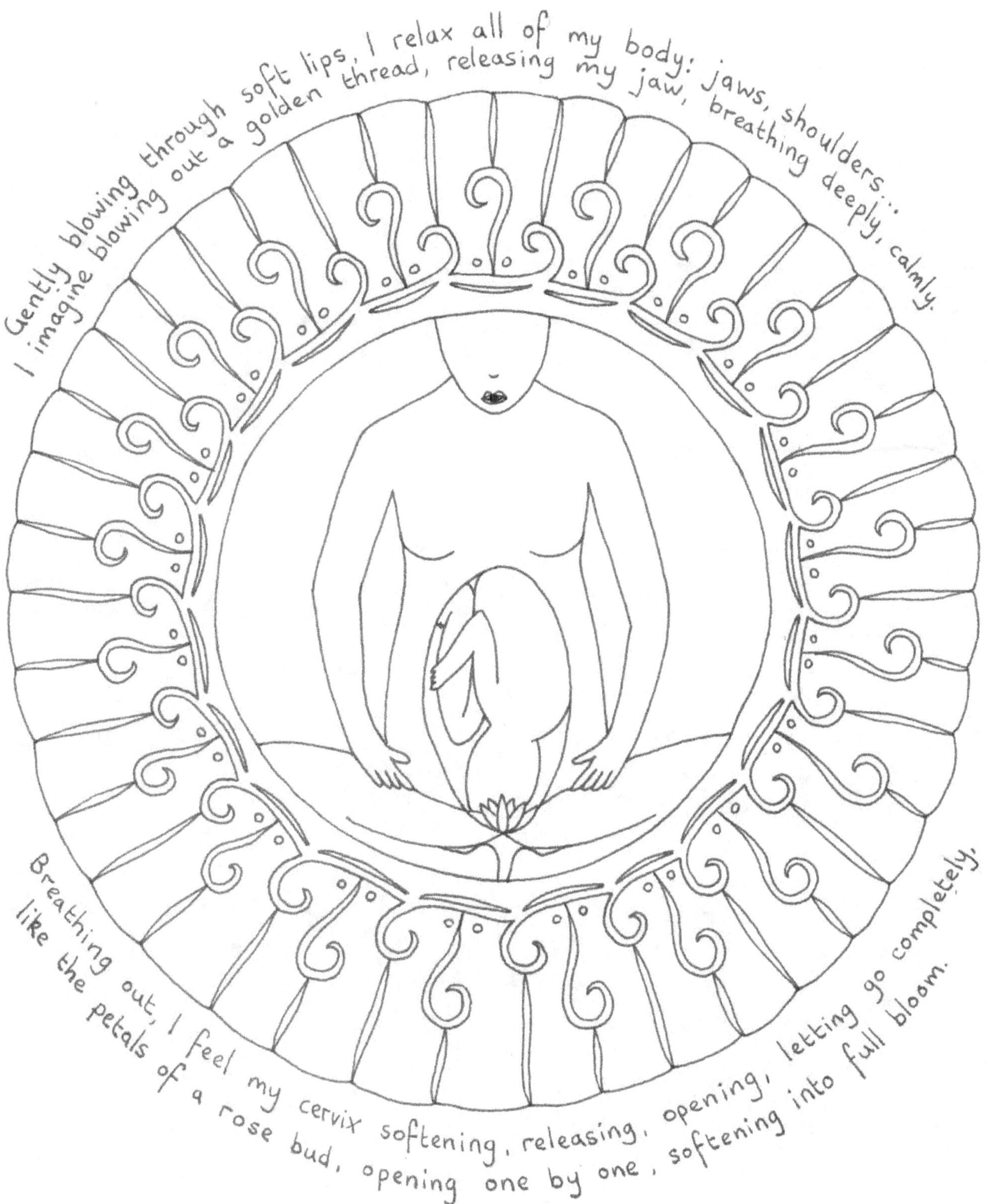

Enjoying pregnancy

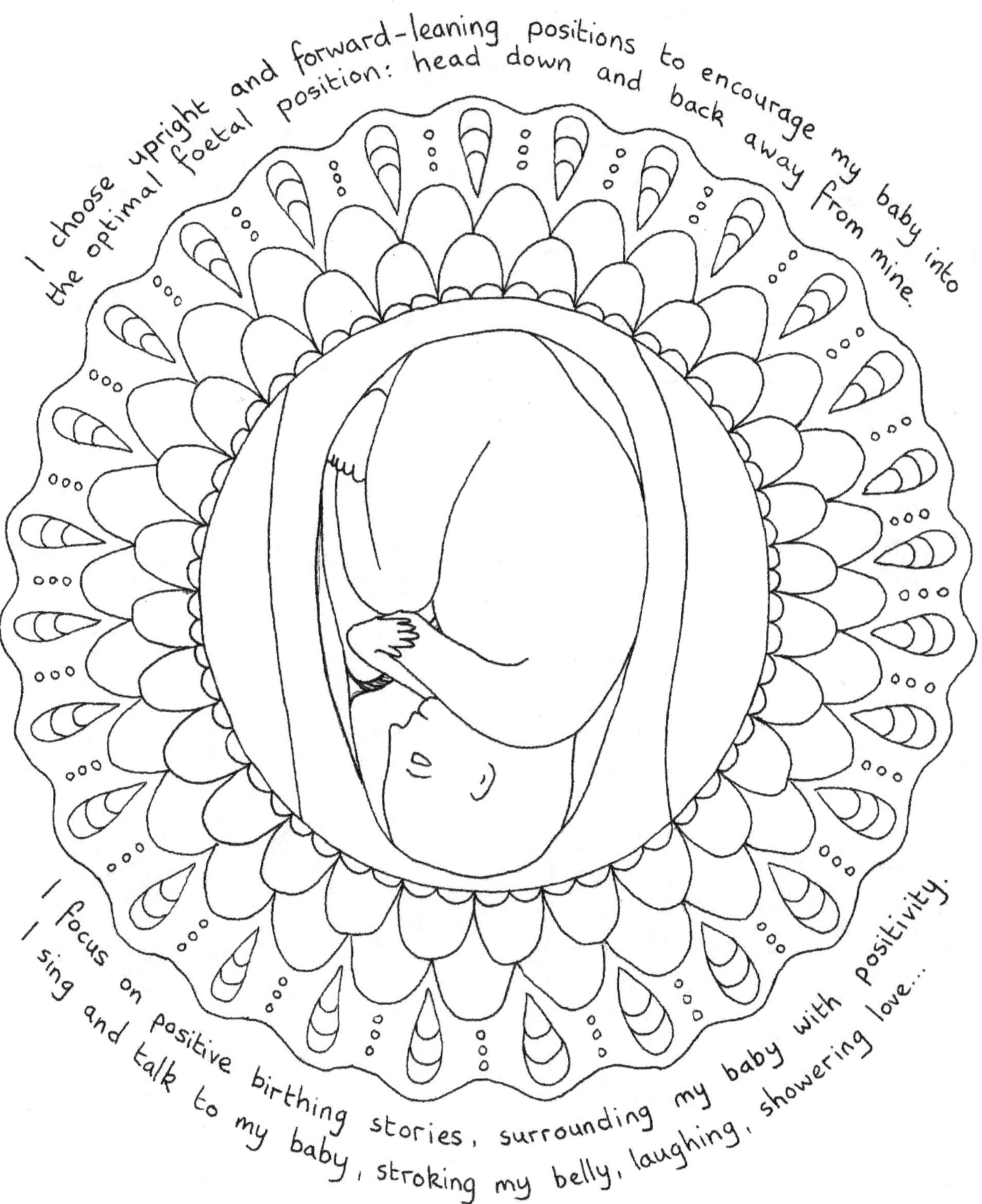

Amazing female anatomy

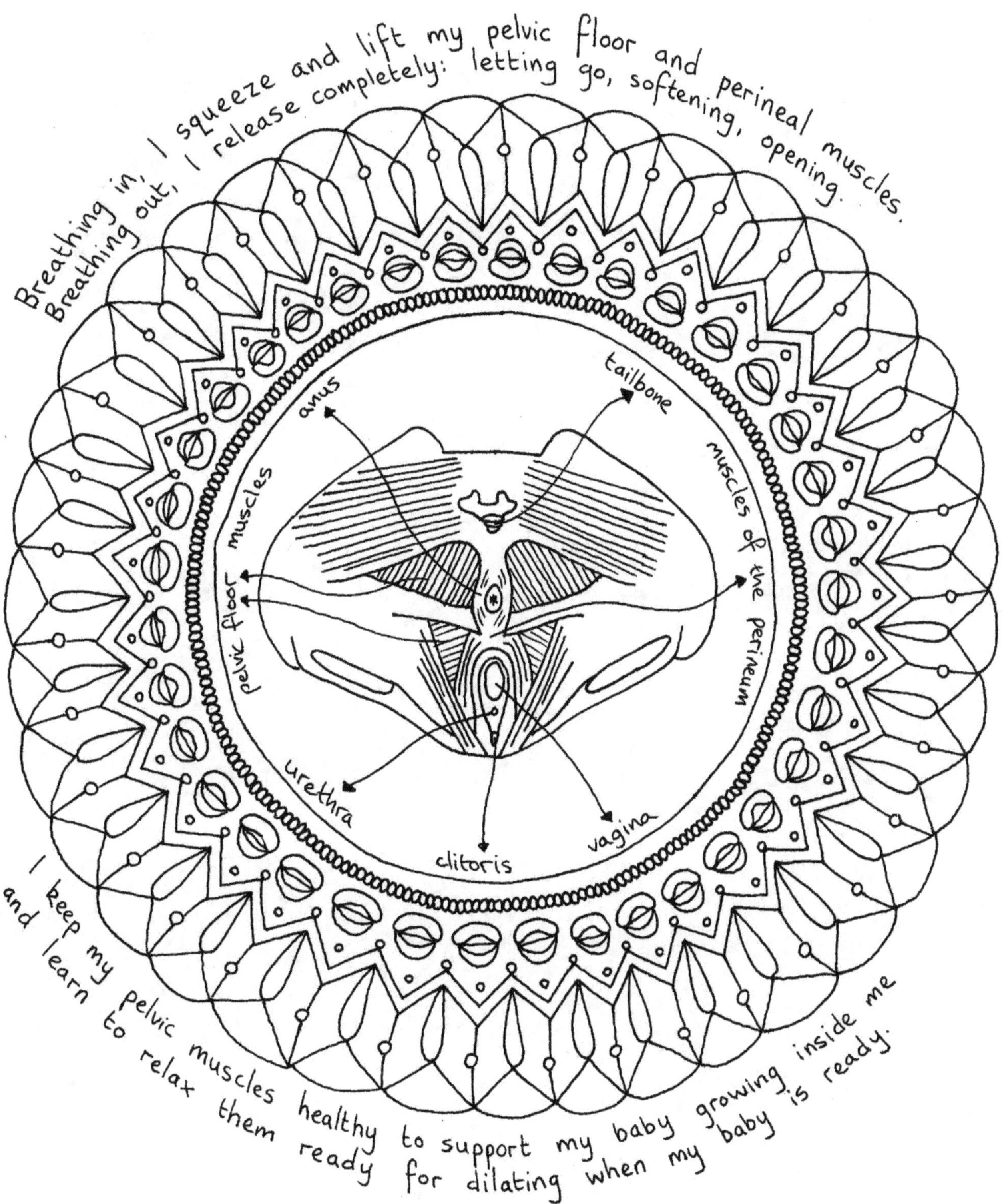

Climbing the mountain

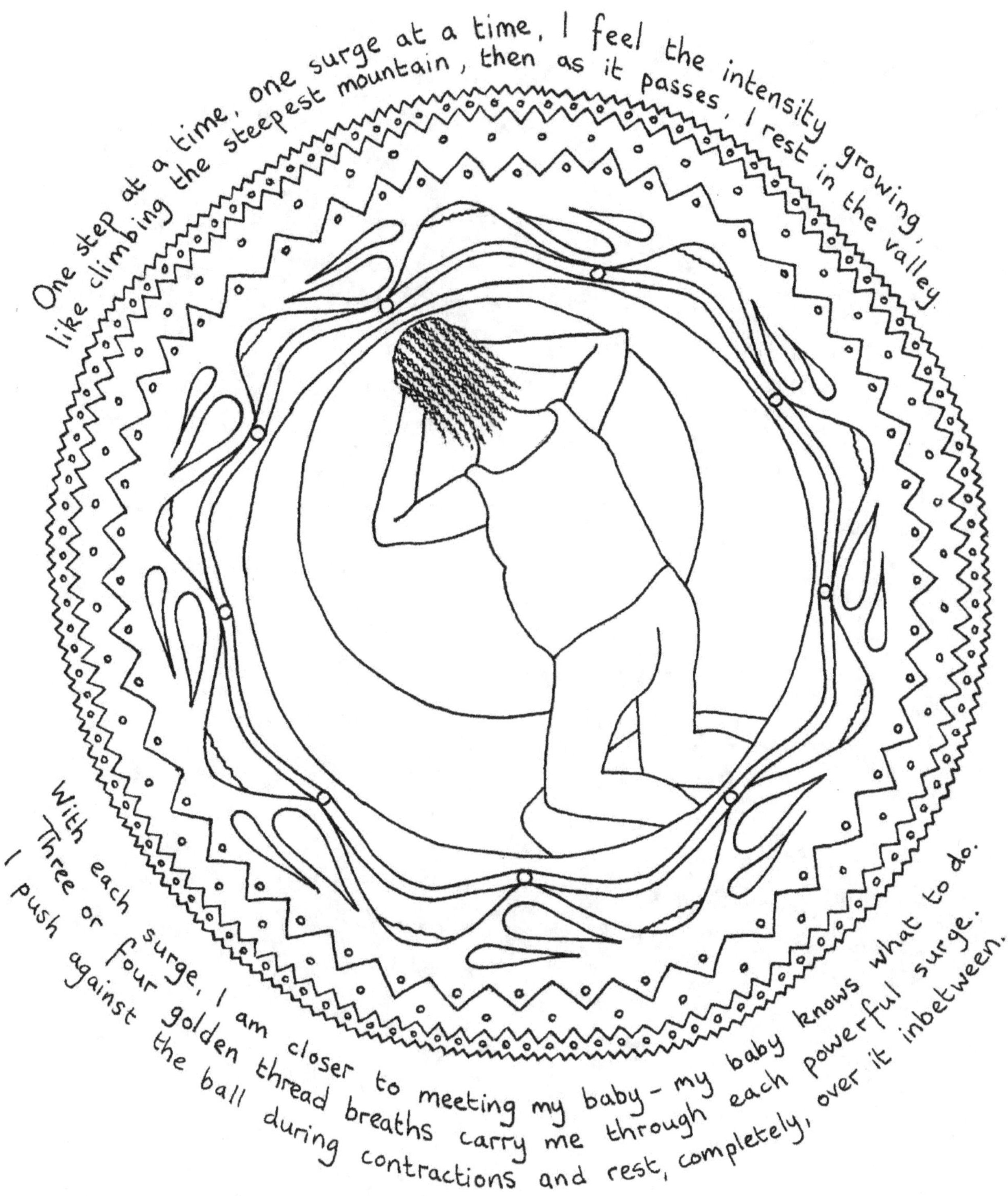

Riding the waves

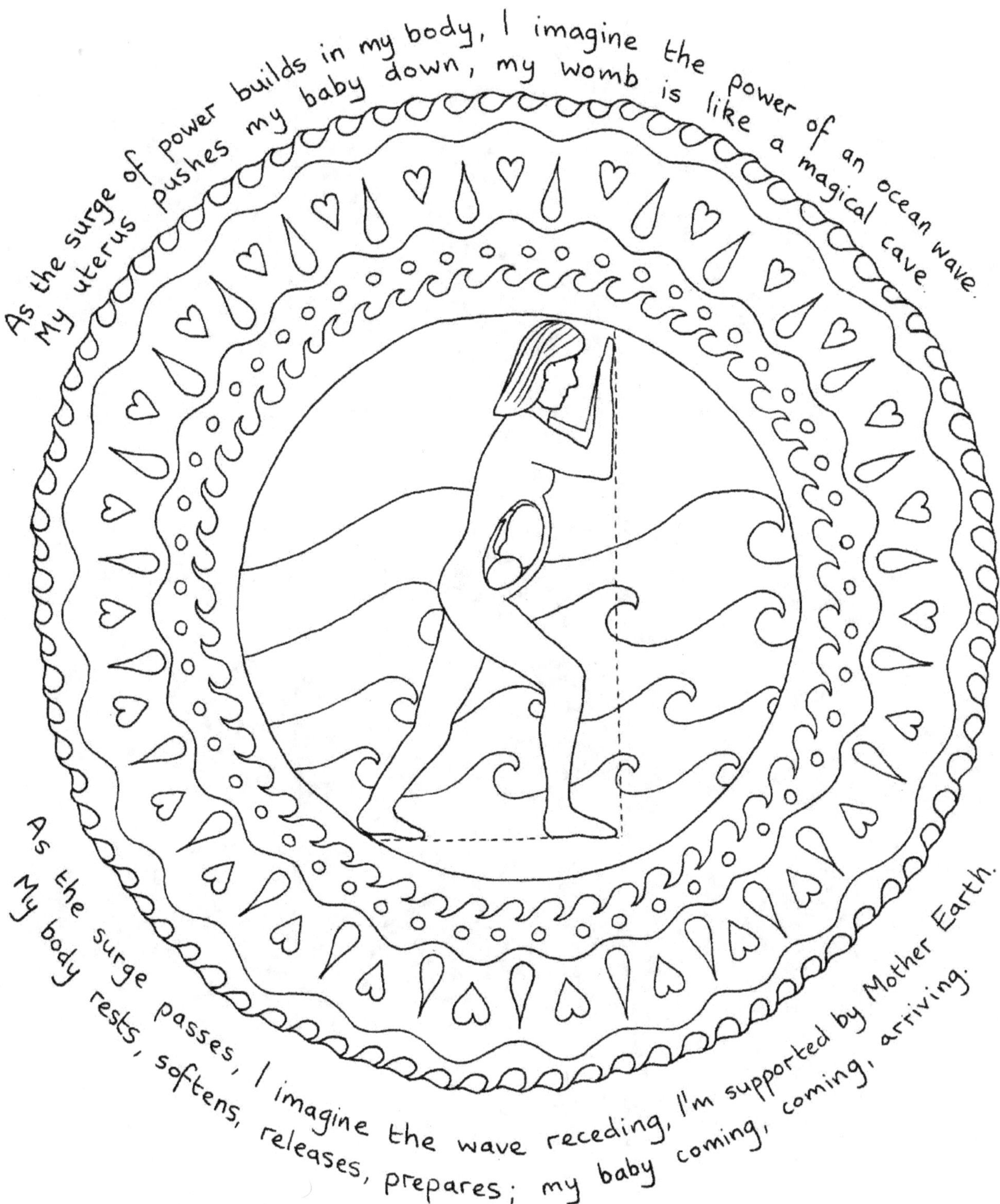

Deeply resting

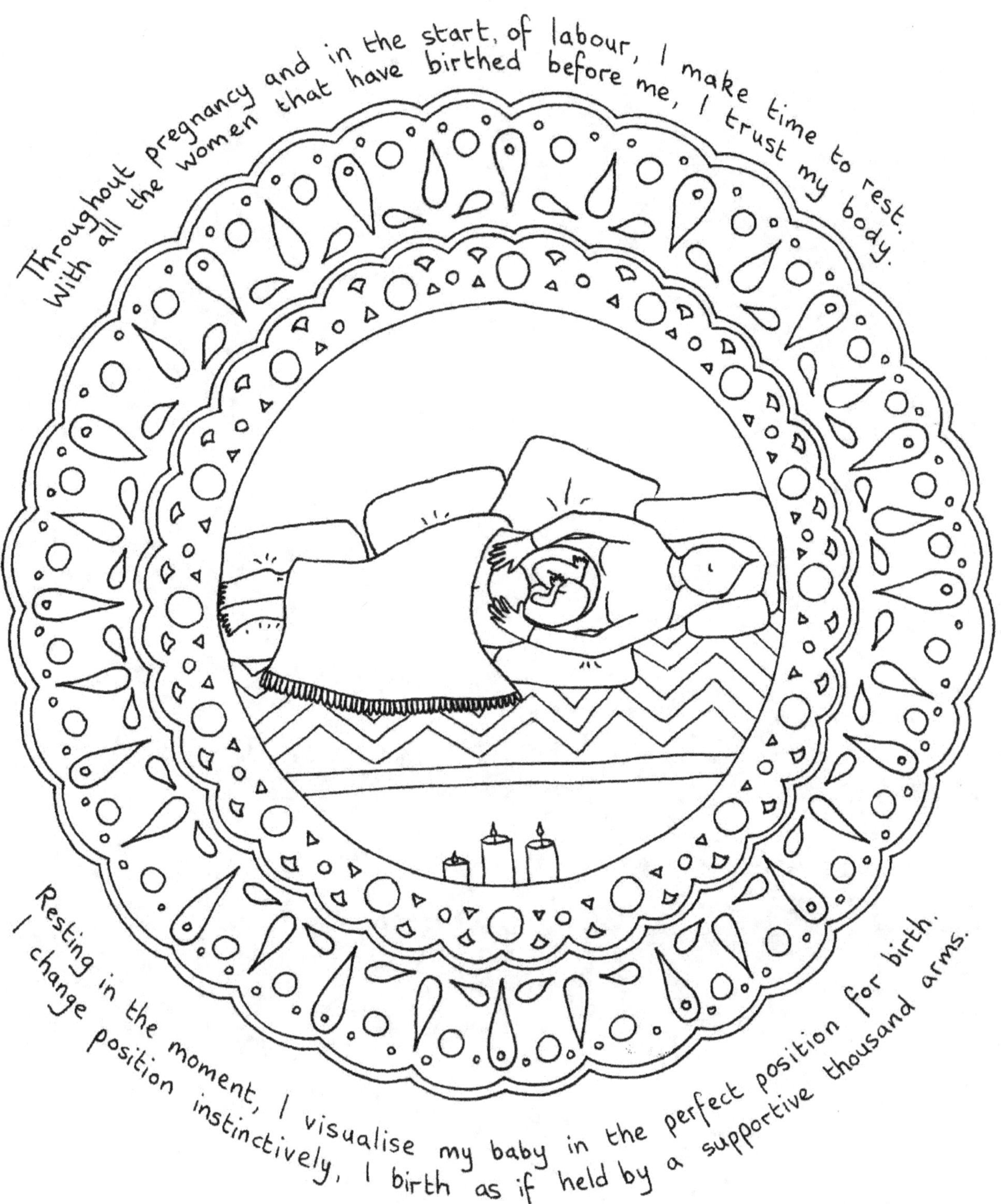

Optimal foetal positioning

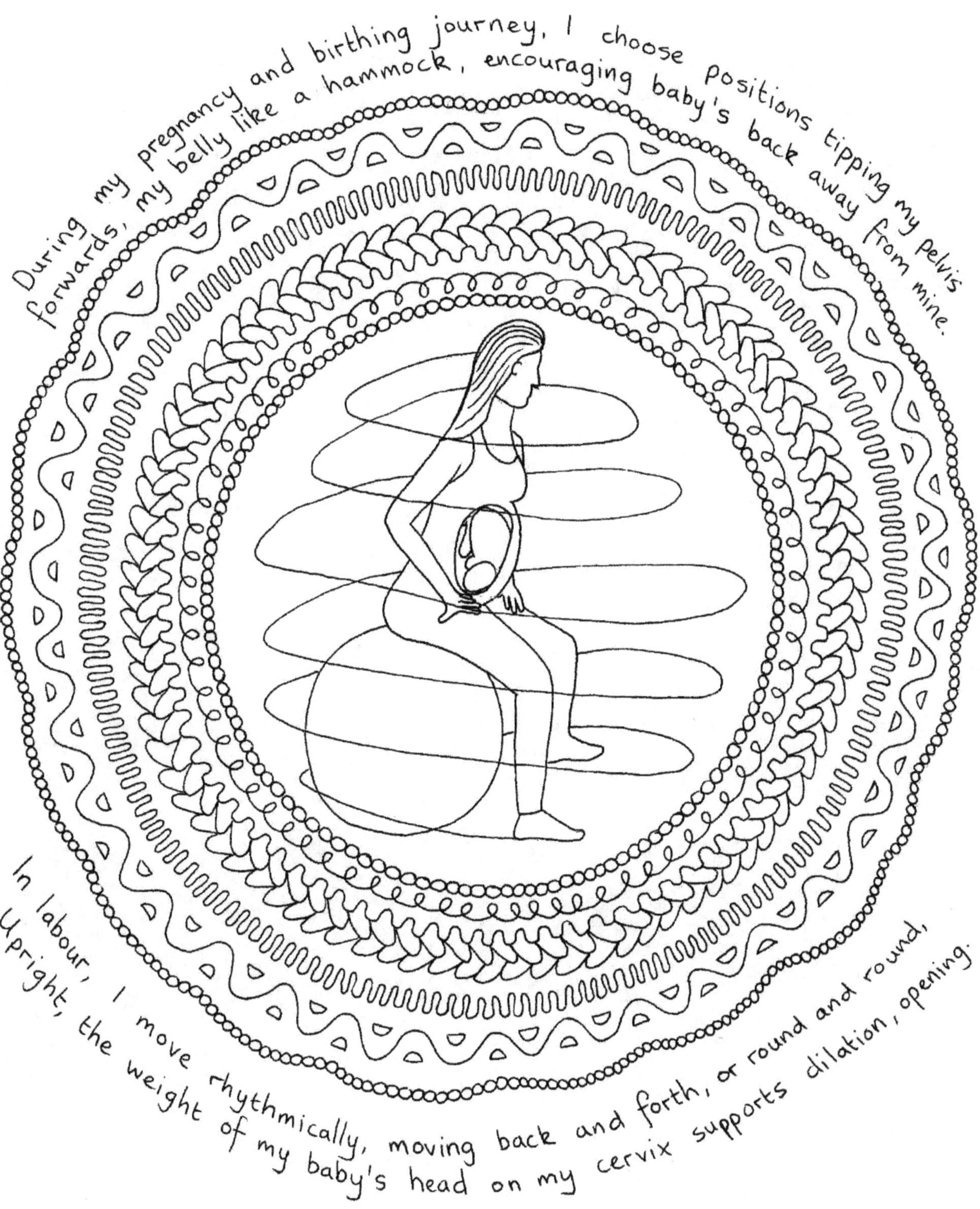

Wonderful water

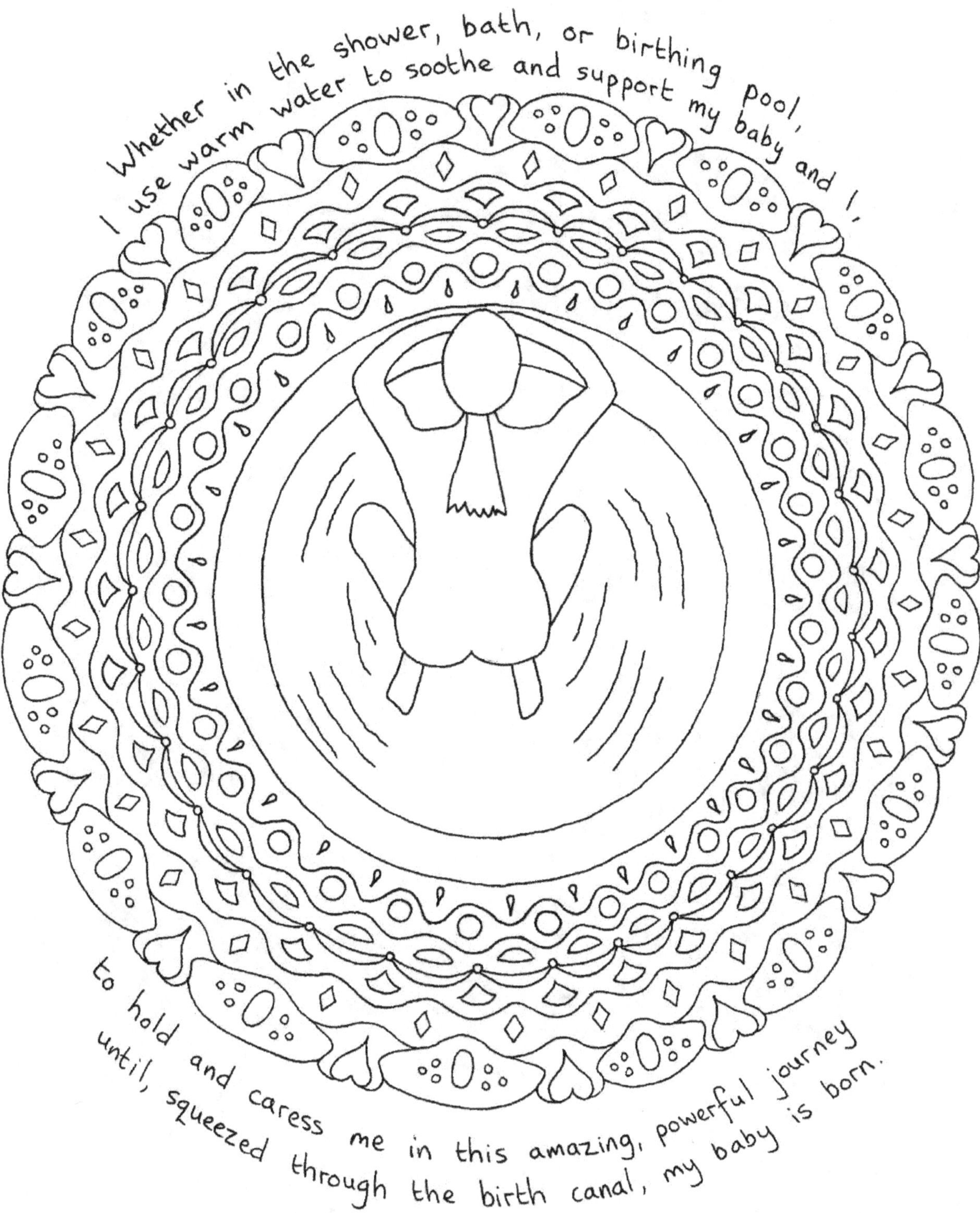

Letting go

As my baby prepares to be born, "I" let go and my body takes over. I let my mind take a back seat, focusing on breathing deeply, calmly.
As I feel my baby's head crowning, I touch the baby's head to believe it. I wait for my body's urge to push, working with the muscular contractions.

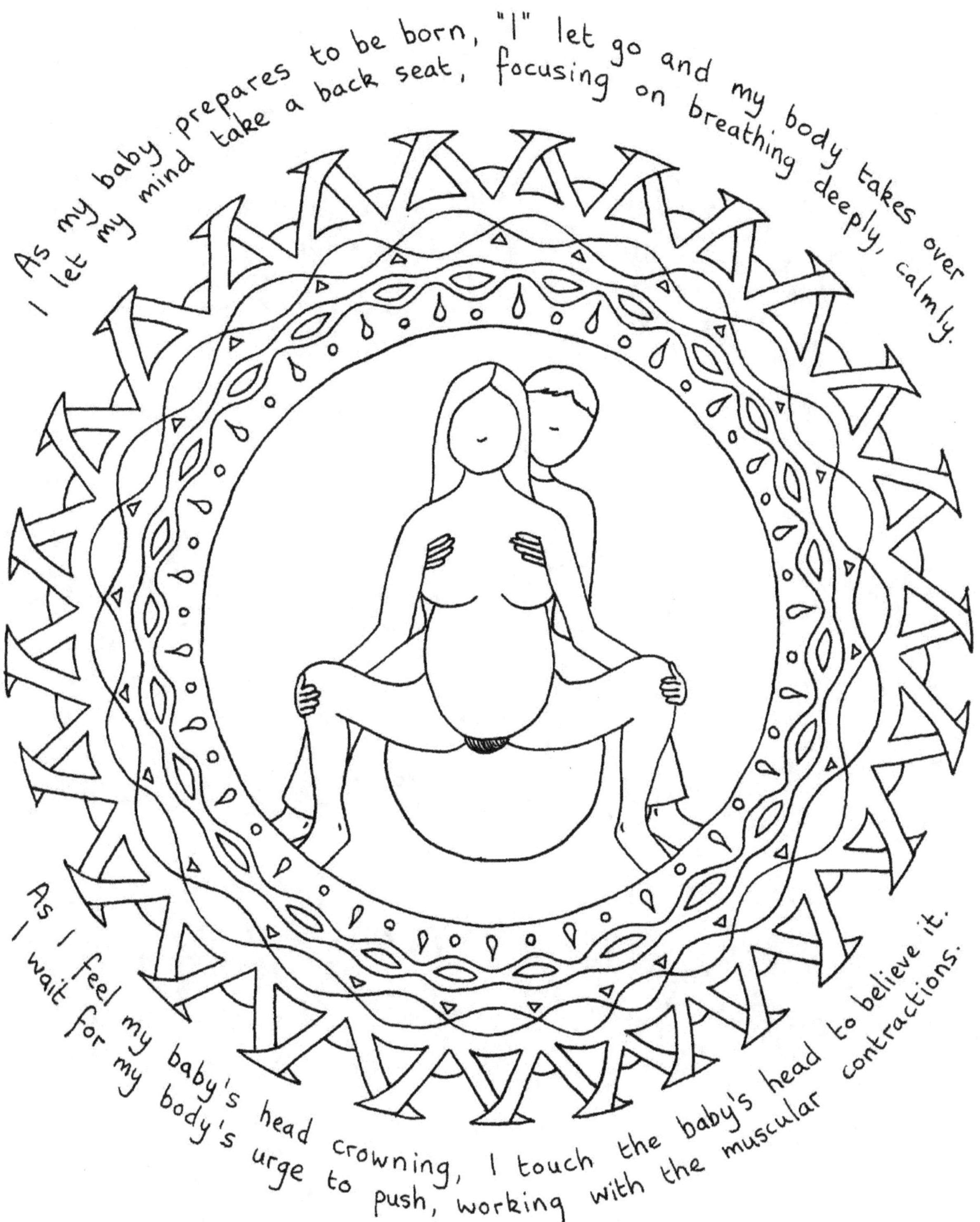

Baby love

So small, so vulnerable, so dependant on me - it can be unnerving
And yet so resilient, this little being, I can't help but be in awe.
Stepping up to this responsibility, this life's work, I give the best of myself.
Within days I know my baby better than anyone, later, the first smile melts my heart.

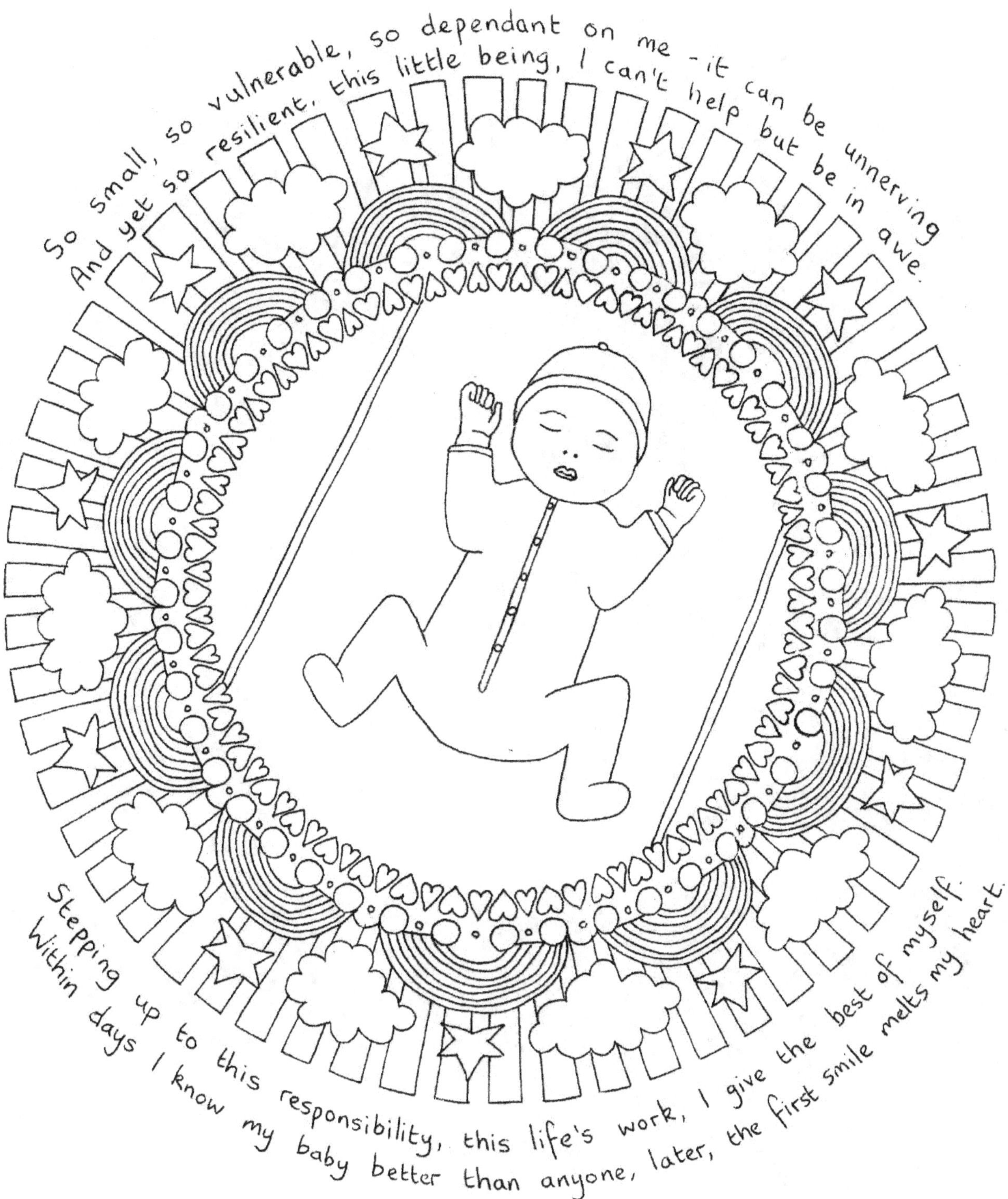

My placenta: the tree of life

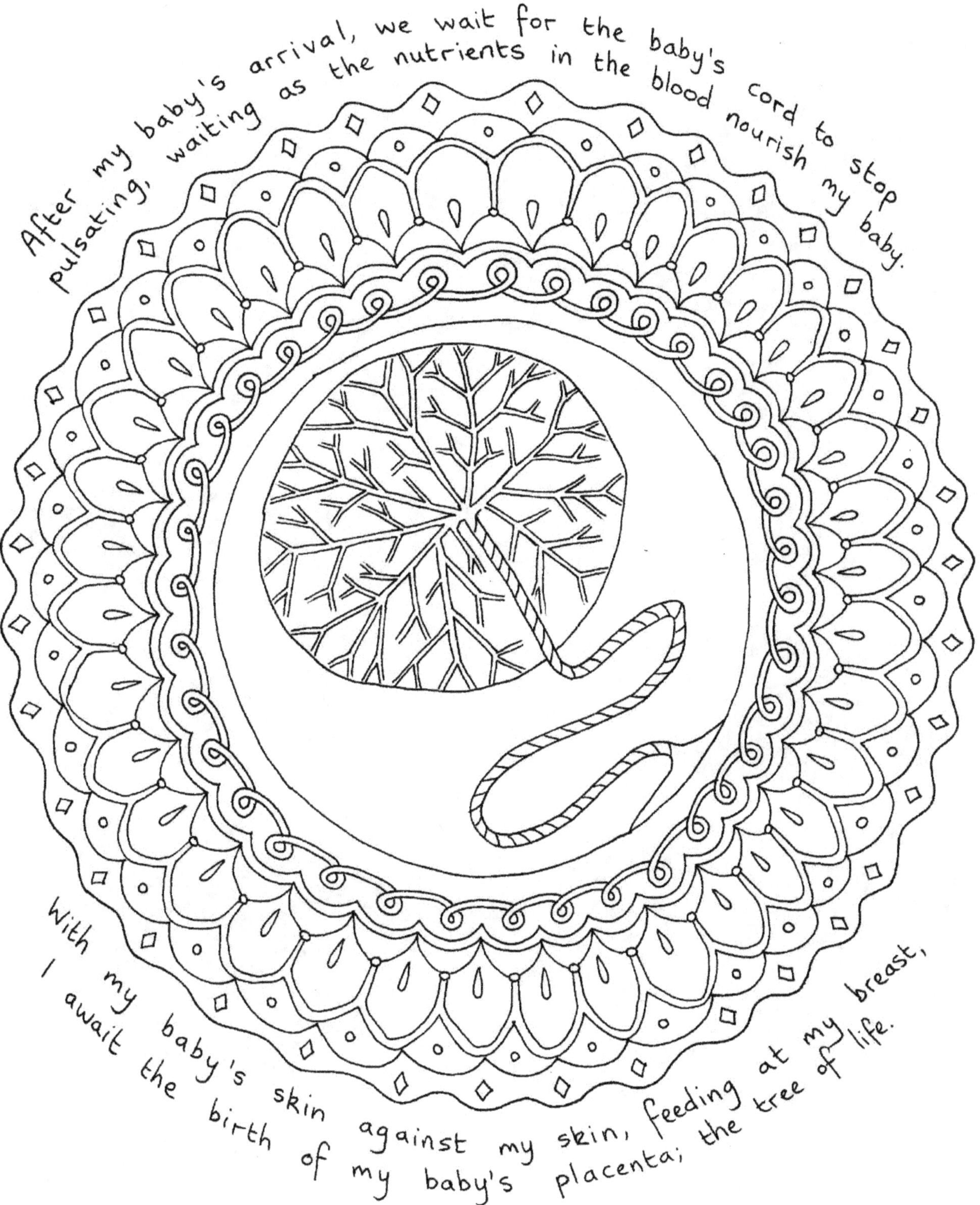

Feeding my baby

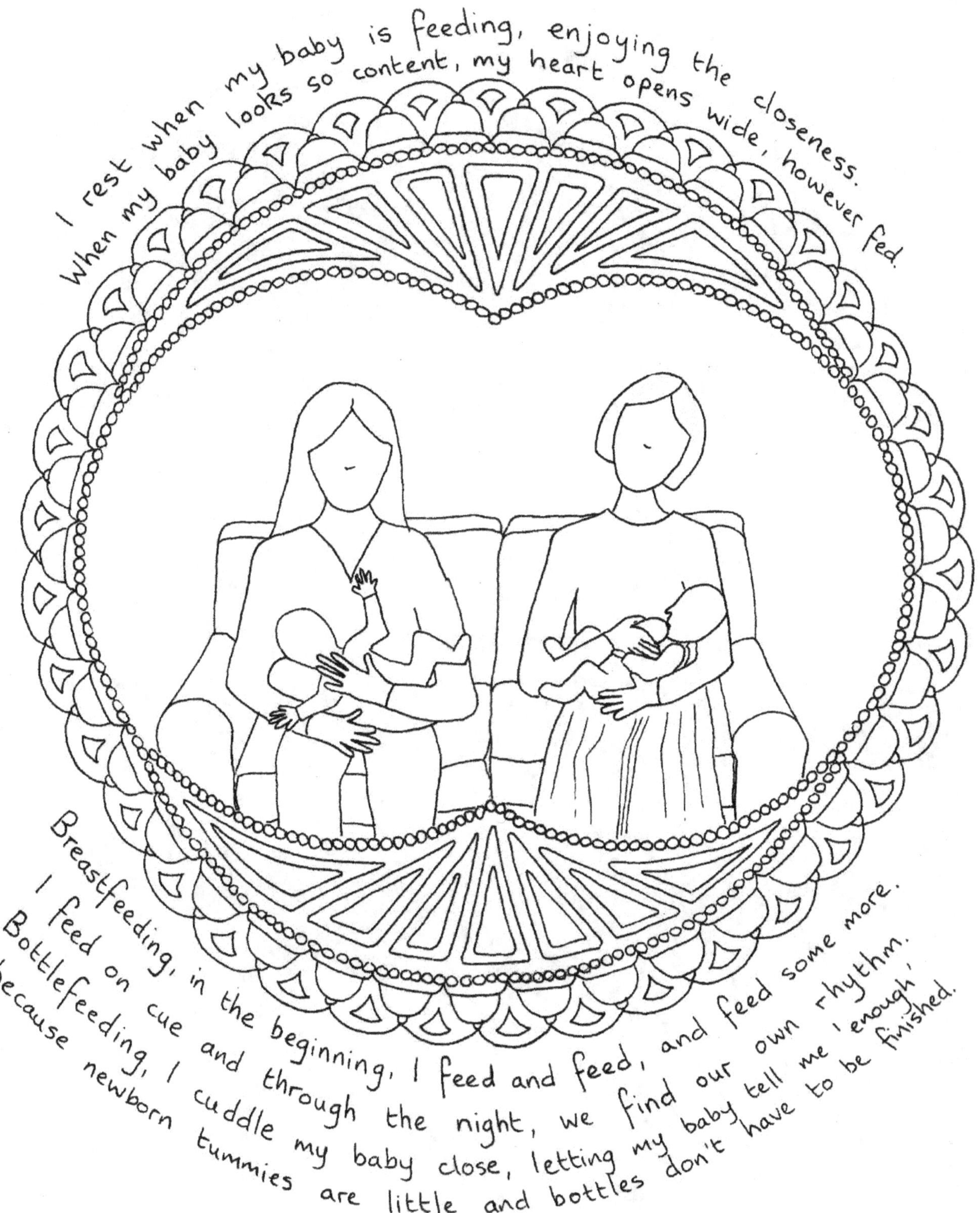

I rest when my baby is feeding, enjoying the closeness.
When my baby looks so content, my heart opens wide, however fed.

Breastfeeding, in the beginning, I feed and feed, and feed some more.
I feed on cue and through the night, we find our own rhythm.
Bottlefeeding, I cuddle my baby close, letting my baby tell me 'enough',
because newborn tummies are little and bottles don't have to be finished.

Growing into motherhood

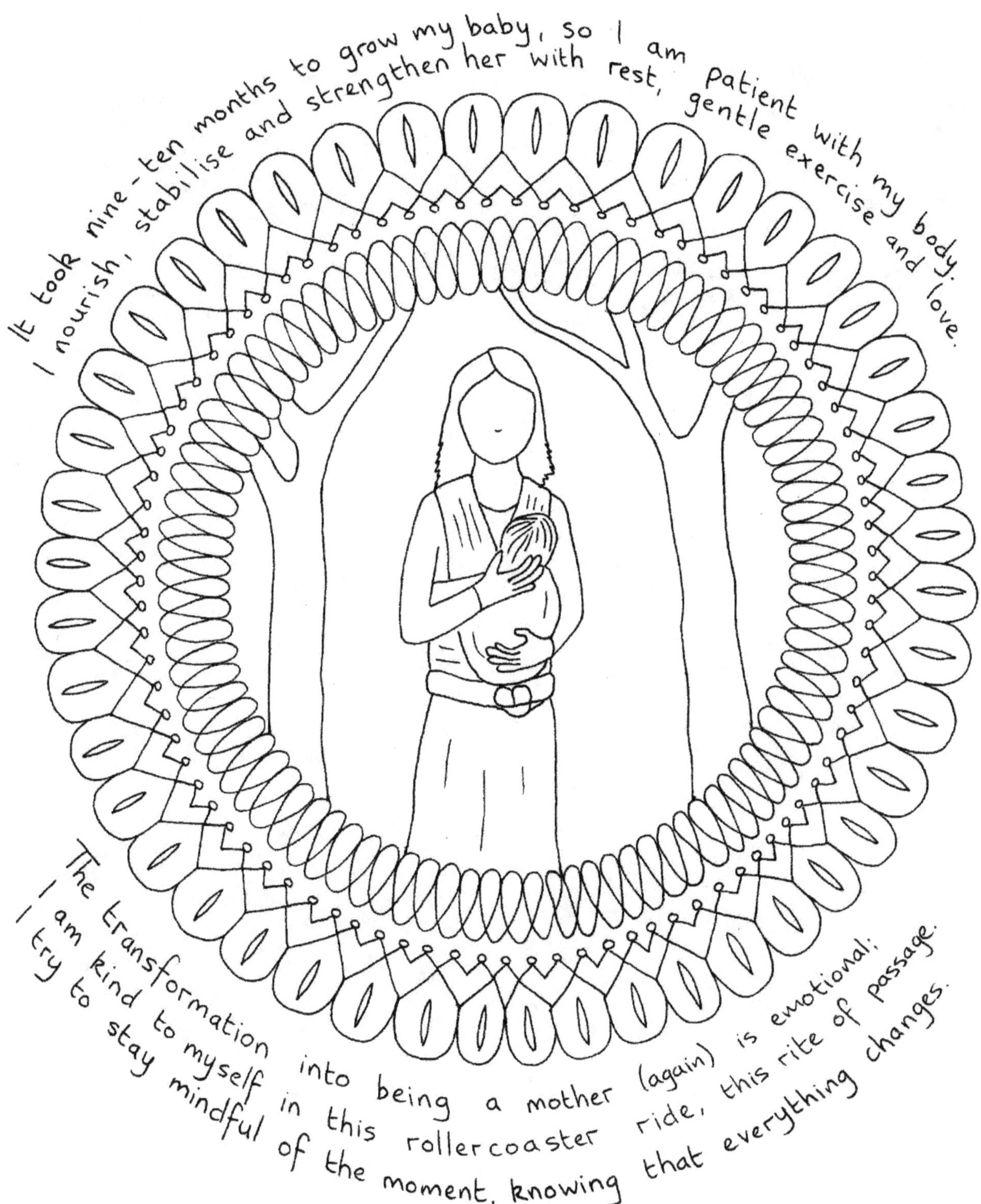

My mandala

You can glue, stick, doodle, squiggle, draw or paint your own...

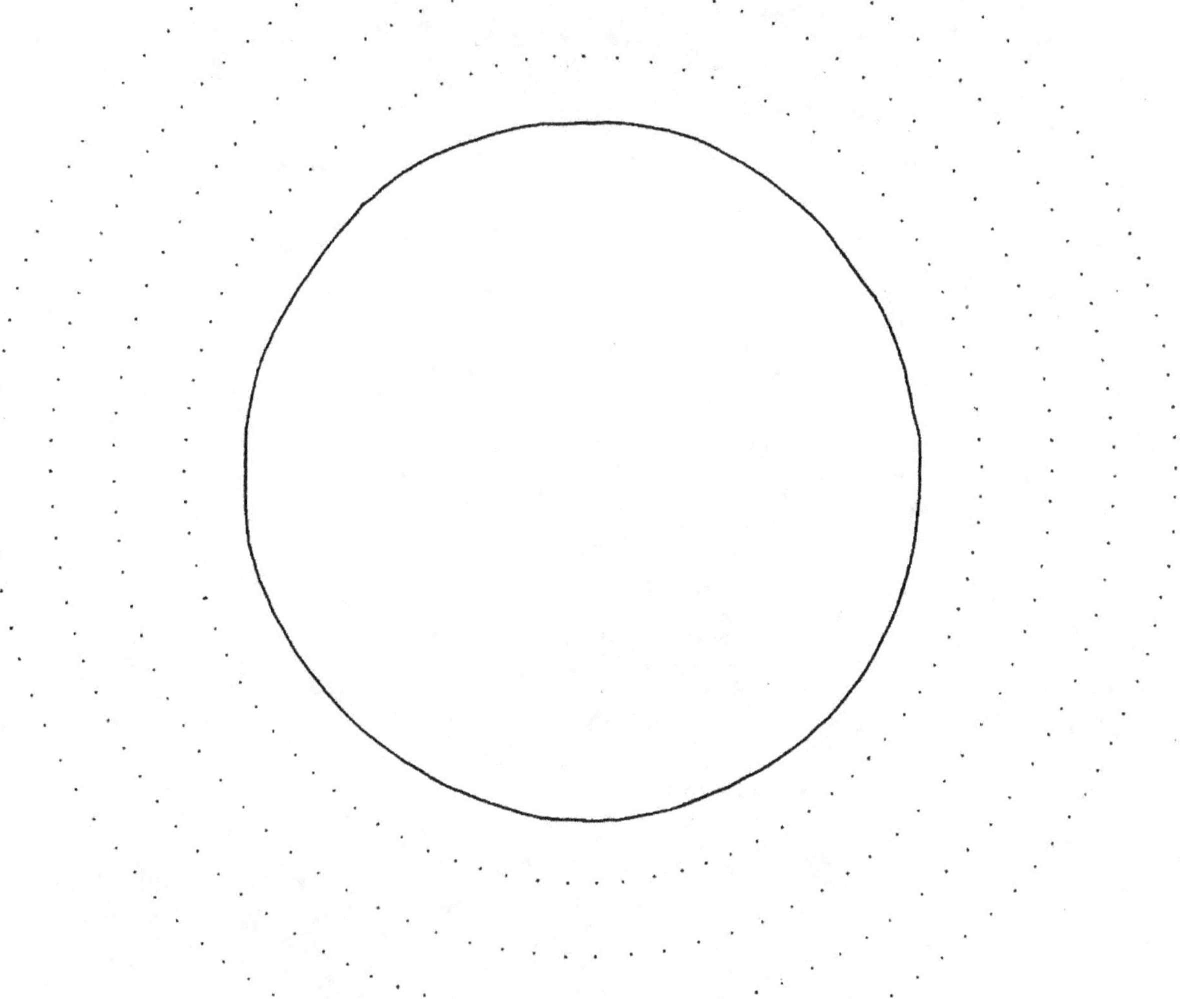

Write your own affirmation: positive and in the present tense ↥

Our birthing story

Write around the spiral, starting at the heart

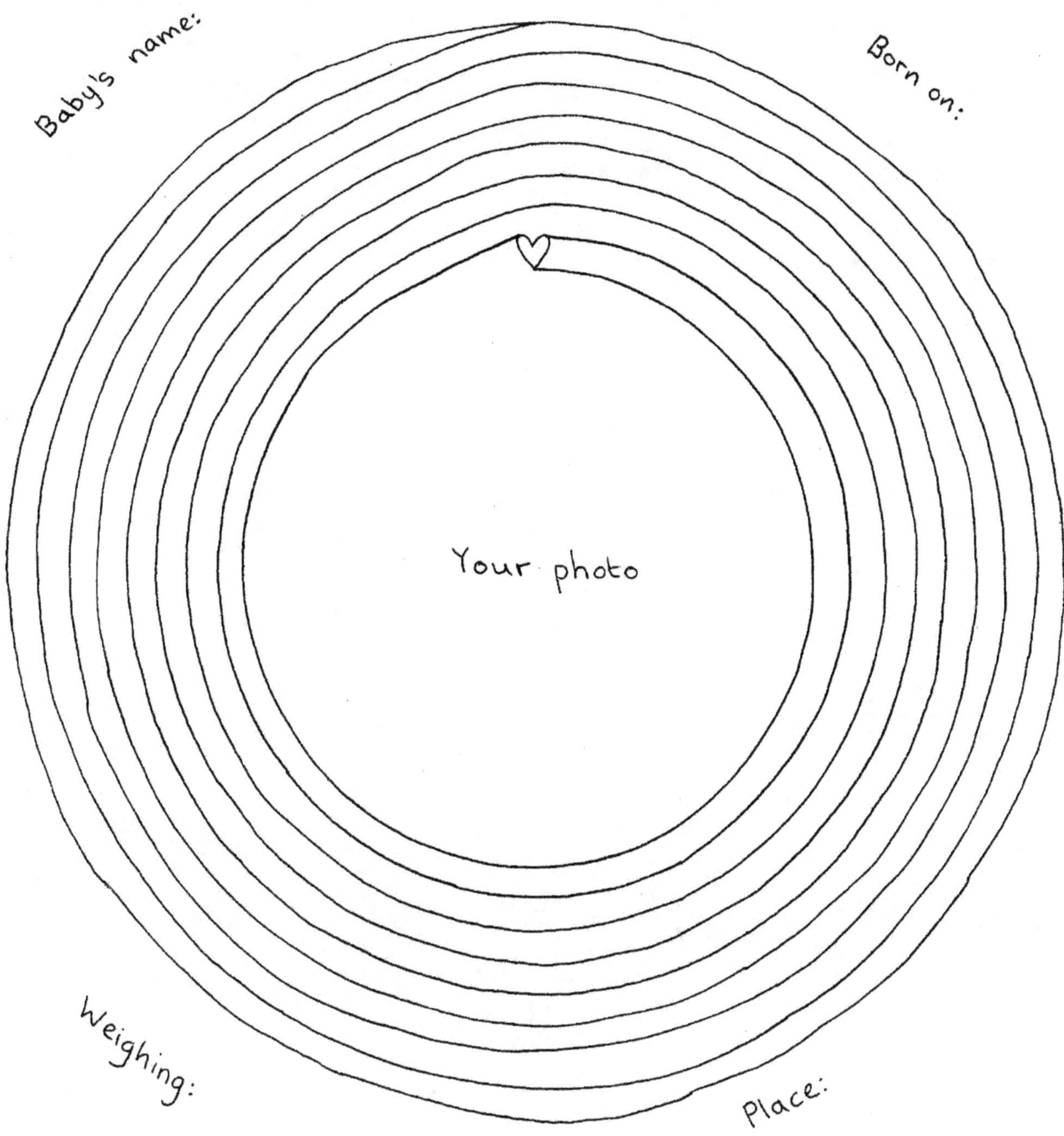

Yoga Nidra instructions

To maximise the benefits of this practice, I suggest choosing the same place to listen to your recording if you can to strengthen the association with relaxation. If you are birthing at home, you could even listen wherever you are planning to birth your baby. It is helpful not to lie on your bed because you are more likely to fall asleep. Instead, choose somewhere that can be your place for Yoga Nidra: quiet and comfort are the most important qualities. If there is only your bed to practice on, change something about how you lie: perhaps, lying with your head where your feet normally are, or with a cushion under your knees to release your lower back.

If you do fall asleep, you will still benefit from the practice. It is quite normal to hear new parts of the Yoga Nidra each time you listen, as your conscious mind focuses at different moments. Please do not listen to a recording when driving.

Positioning

To set yourself up, have a few cushions and a blanket nearby. Lie on your left side and have enough cushions under your head to feel comfortable. There are two options for your legs. You could place cushions, pillows or yoga blocks between your knees and ankles to release any pressure on your pelvis (see picture 1). Alternatively, you can straighten your bottom leg and bend your right knee up so your thigh is about 90° to your body. Then put enough cushions, pillows or yoga blocks under your right knee and foot so that the knee is almost as high as the hip, in order to release pressure on your pelvis or weight through your left hip (picture 2). You could put a folded blanket under your bump.

Picture 1   Picture 2

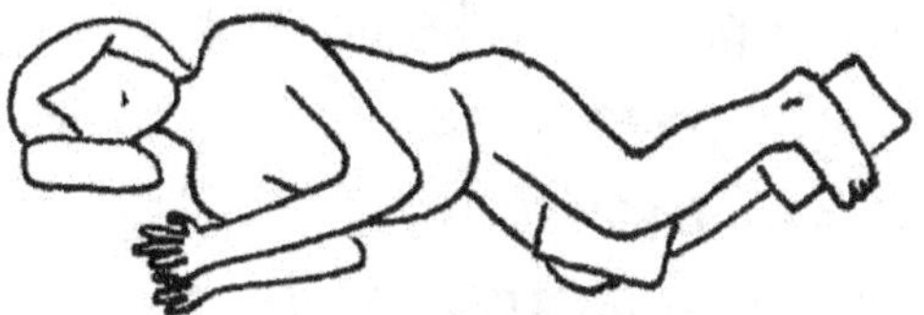

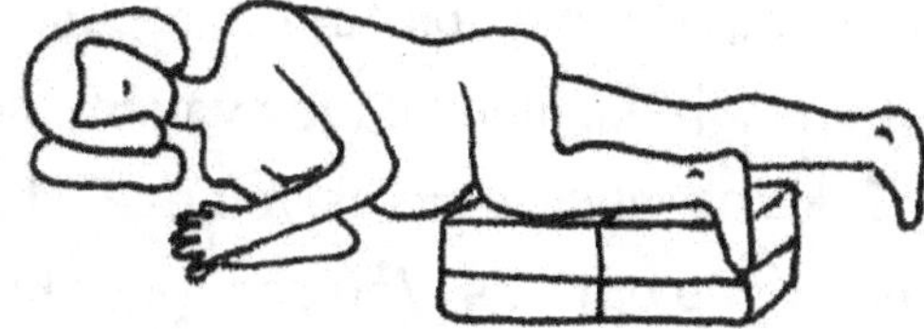

If your birthing partner is listening there are three options. S/he could spoon you with support under the head. Alternatively s/he could lie supine, with the legs straight and the big toes relaxing out to the sides, or with pillows under the knees to release the lower back.

Frequency

I would recommend listening to a Yoga Nidra recording every day if possible. Once you are on maternity leave, you could listen to both tracks each day. However, every time you listen is beneficial and the benefits accumulate over time, so do not worry if every day is not achievable. You could also listen to the recordings during the birthing journey itself, to reinforce your ability to relax through the association with the familiar voice.

Suggestions for recording the scripts

Ensure that there will be quiet and no interruptions while you are recording. Turn off phones and put a note on the front door! Read aloud through the script before recording, so you can understand how it flows and leave appropriately lengthed pauses. Talk slowly and at a consistent pace. Try to use your natural voice, rather than a special relaxing one.

Alternatively, you can access recordings of my voice guiding you through these practices at www.tessayoga.co.uk/colouringbookdownloads

Yoga Nidra script 1: for the pregnant woman & her birthing partner (approx. 15 mins)

Allow yourself to settle in a comfortable position. If you're pregnant, lie on your left side, with enough cushions under your head, bump and top leg to be comfortable. Take as much time as you need to get settled. If you're the partner, you have two options. You can lie behind your pregnant partner, or lie on your back. Make sure you have enough cushions under your head to be comfortable. Wriggle and fidget until you're as settled as can be.

If you are really uncomfortable, perhaps because the baby has changed position, or your hip is aching you can move, but see whether you can move with awareness and return to stillness.

Feel that your body is totally supported. Feel the harder and softer parts of your body against the surface that you are lying on. Feel the clothes against your body and where your skin is open to the air. Begin to release any physical tension that you are holding onto, including releasing the jaw, the shoulders, the hips and buttocks. Now feel that every breath out is helping you settle a little further, resting deeper. *PAUSE.* Every exhalation is giving your body permission to rest deeper and deeper. *PAUSE.*

It can be helpful to set an intention about the pregnancy or birth at the start of the Yoga Nidra practice. Think what your heart's desire in relation to the pregnancy or birth. It might take the form of words, positive, in the present tense. It could be something like: I trust my (or her) body to birth our baby. I trust my (or her) body to birth our baby. Choose words that are meaningful for you. Say it with conviction, like you 100% believe it three times. But you might not have words for your heart's desire, it may be a positive feeling, a picture (like your newborn baby's face) or just an openness to hearing from your heart.

Now I will take your awareness around your body encouraging it to settle more deeply. Take your awareness to the eyebrow centre, imagine a shining light at each point. Then to the throat,

right shoulder, inside of right elbow, inside of right wrist, right thumb, index finger, middle finger, ring finger, little finger, right wrist, right elbow, front of right shoulder,

throat, left shoulder, inside of left elbow, inside left wrist, left thumb, index finger, middle finger, ring finger, little finger, left wrist, left elbow, front left shoulder,

throat, centre of breastbone, left breast, centre of breastbone, right breast, centre of breastbone, navel, pubic bones

right hip bone, right knee, right ankle, right big toe, second toe, third toe, fourth toe, fifth toe, right ankle, right knee, right hip, pubic bones left hip bone, left knee, left ankle, left big toe, second toe, third toe, fourth toe, fifth toe, left ankle, left knee, left hip, pubic bones

navel, centre of breastbone, throat, eyebrow centre.

Now feel that your body is incredibly heavy. You are aware of heaviness in your body from your head to your toes. So heavy, grounded, rooted. Now feel that your body is light, weightless, floating upwards. You feel a wonderful lightness spreading all the way through your body, spacious. Now you sense a coolness throughout your body, feeling as if your body temperature is dropping slightly. You feel a freshness while your body feels so cool. Now you feel a comfortable warmth spreading through your body, from your toes to your head. Now you experience your body as perfect.

Now you can use the golden thread breath. Breathe in through the nostrils and out through soft lips. The lips are just parted and you blow gently out for the length of the exhale, your lips getting softer and softer. Can you imagine a golden thread, fine like gossamer, being blown out, releasing the jaw? In through the nostrils, and blowing out through soft lips. Let your breath be relaxed and easeful. *PAUSE.* Now as you breathe in, count 9; exhale fully blowing out the golden thread, and as you breathe in again count 8. Each inhalation counting down toward 0. It's fine if you need to come back to 9 and start again. *(Pause while counting down, allowing enough time for 9 breaths.)*

Now you can imagine, if you like, your baby. Safely snuggled inside, being nourished, developing moment to moment by the amazing female body. You are making space in your life for the baby to arrive and be part of your family. You are slowing down, nesting, preparing for becoming a parent for the first (or second or third) time. You know that the baby is developing without any conscious direction and that the female body works perfectly to support your baby. You know that birth is a natural process. You can feel a deep trust in the female body to protect and nourish your baby. You deeply trust the female body instinctively knows how to birth your baby.

During the birthing journey, you follow your instincts. The birthing woman moving instinctively into whatever positions are comfortable. The birthing partner models how to breathe deeply, reminding her to breathe deeply. You both know that resting and being calm supports the baby and baby's birth. The birthing woman, the birthing partner and your baby have all the resources they need inside, already there. You can ask for anything that you don't have. You are supported. You are confident, reassured, and positive about the birth. *PAUSE.*

Now take your awareness to hollow at the base of your throat, between your collarbones. Then as you breathe in, take your awareness to the base of the throat. As you breathe out, drop your awareness down to your baby or your navel. As you breathe in, travel up to the base of your throat, as you breathe out, travel down to your baby in the womb or your navel. It is as if you have a little two way telescope so that you can see your baby, and your baby can see you. PAUSE. Feel that every time you breathe out, you let go, let go let go, so that only positive feelings remain. Every time you breathe in, you deepen the connection with your baby. *PAUSE.*

Return to your intention about the pregnancy or birth. Think what your heart's desire is, in relation to the pregnancy or birth. You might repeat words, such as I trust my body to birth my baby, or remember a particular feeling or simply have an openness to your heart's guidance. *PAUSE.*

Now return to the golden thread breath. Let it carry you back as we come towards the end of the practice. Breathing a little more deeply, feel that as you breathe in, you draw energy into your body. As you blow out the golden thread, or sigh, or yawn, you are re-connecting with the world around you. *PAUSE.*

Be aware of any sounds in the room and outside of the room. Follow them back as you come towards the end of the practice.

Become aware of your body lying down, resting. Now you feel ready to move, wriggling your fingers and toes, then moving your wrists and ankles. You might want to stretch or move in a particular way after being still for a while. You might like to rub your pregnant belly with your hand.

When you are ready to sit up, use your hands or forearms to push up. You might want to eat or drink something. Make sure you are fully alert whilst carrying the benefits of the relaxation into the rest of your day.

The practice of Yoga Nidra has now finished. My best wishes go with you.

Yoga Nidra script 2: for the pregnant woman (approx. 25 mins)

Allow yourself to settle in a comfortable position. Lie on your left side, with enough cushions under your head, bump and top leg to be comfortable. Take as much time as you need to get settled. Make any adjustments so you are as comfortable as possible.

If you are really uncomfortable, perhaps because the baby has changed position, or your hip is aching, you can move, but see whether you can move with awareness and return to stillness.

Now feel that you are settling your body against the earth. Wherever you are lying, feel that your body wants to settle on the ground, to feel rooted, earthed and grounded. Every breath out, you settle a little more, almost as if you could leave a mark on the ground, held and cradled by Mother Earth. Every exhalation, resting a little deeper. *PAUSE.*

Now as you breathe, feel your breath flowing like water in and out of your body. Whether it's through your mouth or your nostrils, feel the breathing flowing effortlessly, so easefully, so comfortably. The breath flows into the body, trickling into any nooks and crannies in the body that need to let go a little more. Every inhalation, feeling a little lighter and more buoyant. *PAUSE.*

Now feel or imagine your baby inside your womb, inside your amazing body. You can imagine, if you like, all the nutrients passing through the placenta and through the umbilical cord to your baby, supporting your baby. All the energy from the wholesome food that you are eating is nourishing your baby. Your baby feels you settling into this relaxation, feels a wonderful relaxed energy surrounding him or her. You sense the warmth your baby creates, nestled safely within you. *PAUSE.*

Now you become aware of your heart, and feel there the love and other positive feelings that you have about your baby. Like a gentle breeze, you imagine or feel those feelings drifting towards your baby, encircling him or her in these wonderful positive feelings. You know that your baby hears the sound of your breath whooshing in and out of the lungs, the sound of your voice when you speak or sign to him or her. *PAUSE.*

Now you become aware of the space in your body that you have created for your baby to grow, and the space in your heart that you have created to love your baby, and space in your life to welcome your baby into your family. You find a spaciousness in your body even as your baby gets bigger, you wonder at how magnificent your body is to transform to grow your baby.

It can be helpful to set an intention about the pregnancy or birth at the start of the Yoga Nidra practice. Think what your heart's desire is, in relation to the pregnancy or birth. It might take the form of words, positive, in the present tense. It could be something like: I trust my (or her) body to birth our baby. I trust my (or her) body to birth our baby. Choose words that are meaningful for you. Say it with conviction, like you 100% believe it three times. But you might not have words for your heart's desire, it may be a positive feeling, a picture (like your newborn baby's face) or just an openness to hearing from your heart. PAUSE.

You feel that you are in a place of safety and wellness. I will take you around your body, encouraging each part to rest more deeply. Being here is enough, listening is enough, there is nothing more that you need to do. You can imagine, if you like a gentle caress on each part that I mention. Take your awareness to the eyebrow centre. Then to the throat,

right shoulder, inside of right elbow, inside of right wrist, right thumb, index finger, middle finger, ring finger, little finger, right wrist, right elbow, front of right shoulder,

throat, left shoulder, inside of left elbow, inside left wrist, left thumb, index finger, middle finger, ring finger, little finger, left wrist, left elbow, front left shoulder,

throat, centre of breastbone, left breast, centre of breastbone, right breast, centre of breastbone, navel, pubic bones

right hip bone, right knee, right ankle, right big toe, second toe, third toe, fourth toe, fifth toe, right ankle, right knee, right hip, pubic bones

left hip bone, left knee, left ankle, left big toe, second toe, third toe, fourth toe, fifth toe, left ankle, left knee, left hip, pubic bones

navel, centre of breastbone, throat, eyebrow centre.

Feel that you are in a place of wellness and safety.

Bring your awareness to your heart, and imagine a tiny golden seed within. As you breathe in, imagine the golden seed expanding out in every direction to become a huge golden sphere far beyond your body. As you breathe out, imagine it condensing back into a tiny golden seen within your heart space. Inhaling, expanding, radiant. Exhaling, condensing, centred. Imagine the golden sphere, as you breathe in, as a protective space for you, just as your womb protects your baby. Feel the golden light connecting you to your baby, protecting your baby. Inhaling, expanding, radiant. Exhaling, condensing, centred. Alternate between these images or words as you breathe. Inhaling, expanding, radiant. Exhaling, condensing, centred. How would it be to be both radiant and centred at the same time? How would that feel? *PAUSE.*

Now let go of those feelings. You can imagine, if you like, that you are a little animal that likes to burrow, perhaps a little rabbit. As you breathe in, you put your head outside the burrow and are alert, curious, checking that everything is safe and secure. As you breathe out, you slip back inside the warm, cosy, safe burrow and feeling totally at home and relaxed. Breathing in, you check that everything is safe. Breathing out, you feel totally at home. Alternative between these feelings or words as you breathe. How would it be to be both checking that everything is safe and feeling totally at home at the same time? How would that feel? *PAUSE.* During your birthing journey you can allow a need to check that everything is safe, whilst being deeply at home in your body and trusting your body to birth your baby? *PAUSE.*

Now you can use the golden thread breath. Breathe in through the nostrils and out through the lips. The lips slightly parted and blowing gently out for the length of the exhale. Can you imagine a golden thread, fine like gossamer, being blown out, releasing the jaw? In through the nostrils, and blowing out through the lips. Let your breath be relaxed and easeful. Now as you breathe in, count 9; exhale fully blowing out the golden thread, and as you breathe in again count 8. Each inhalation counting down toward 0; you are going into "the zone". It's fine if you need to come back to 9 and start again. *(Pause while counting down, watching person with middle length breath.)*

Now let go of the counting, and breathe between the centre of the heart space, behind the breastbone, and down to your baby in your womb. Breathing in, up to the centre of the heart space and breathing out, down to your baby or your navel. In, to the heart, and out, to your baby. PAUSE

As you breathe out, feel that you are gently connecting with your baby (*PAUSE for next breath out:*) As you breathe out, feel that the mind is at rest and your body is functioning perfectly. The mind and the body are completely integrated and connected. (*PAUSE for next breath out:*) As you breathe out, you feel that the mind is at ease, the mind is calm, while the body works efficiently and perfectly. *PAUSE.* As you next breathe out, you feel that the heart is sending love, and gratitude for carrying and nourishing your baby. (*PAUSE for next breath out:*) As you breathe out, you feel that the heart is sending love and gratitude for birthing your baby smoothly when the time is right. *PAUSE.*

You can imagine, if you like, that your baby has decided it's time to come into the world. You feel the muscular contractions of your womb as surges of power that are working smoothly and efficiently to dilate your cervix and open your body, a spacious gateway to allow your baby to be born. You experience these surges of power that are moving your baby down and into the world beyond the womb. Although it's strong, hard work, if it gets too strong, you can breathe through it and change position. *PAUSE.*

You change position instinctively to whatever feels comfortable. You might want to lie on your left side, or lean onto a birthing ball, or push against the wall, or sway, or gently walk. You do what feels good to you. Your baby is communicating with you to tell you how to make room for him or her to move into the best position to be born. You feel safe and protected, you birth as if held by a thousand loving supportive arms, trusting in your body because of all the women that have birthed naturally and joyously before you. *PAUSE.*

As you start your birthing journey begin, you rest, conserving your energy. Using the golden thread breath, you breathe in through the nostrils, bring oxygen to your baby and to your womb. As you blow out between soft lips, you release your jaw and all the way down through the centre of your body to below your baby. You imagine a little flower bud, just below your baby. Every exhalation, you blow the thin golden thread between the lips, and feel or imagine the flower petals peeling away one at a time, softening, opening, release until the flower is in full bloom. Every breath, every surge of power, bringing you closer to meeting your baby. You gently focus on opening and softening, letting go, letting go, letting go. *PAUSE.*

As the surge builds in your womb, you imagine the power of an ocean wave. This wave of energy is helping your baby to come into the world. These surges of power are your friend; you want a strong and powerful friend to help you in this physical journey. Your womb is like a magical cave, protecting your baby. When the time is right, the waves wash into the cave and safely, smoothly bring your baby down and out into the world. As each surge passes, you imagine the wave receding, soothing, calming. Your body rests completely. You rest completely. Your mind focused within your body, on this amazing birthing journey. You feel your feet on solid ground, supported by Mother Earth. PAUSE

As the surge buildings in your womb, you imagine climbing a safe, solid mountain. Your body is working hard, functioning perfectly. Then you reach the peak of the surge, and the peak of the safe, solid mountain and can see the view: looking ahead to when your baby will be in your arms. You go down the other side of the mountain, to rest in the valley. All the time you are breathing deeply, using the golden thread breath. You might focus on three or four golden thread breaths to carry you through one surge as the birthing journey progresses. Your body rests completely. You rest completely. Your mind focused within your body, on this amazing birthing journey. You feel your feet on solid ground, supported by Mother Earth. *PAUSE.*

You allow yourself to be supported and guided through this birthing journey, both by the people around you and with your own natural resources. You let go, let go, let go. In birthing your baby, you are also being reborn into a new phase of your life. You let go, let go, let go. You are in a place of safety and wellness. *PAUSE.*

You let your mind rest deeply, gently focused only on the breath and the waves of your body working. Your mind rests while your body works effectively, functions perfectly to birth your baby smoothly. When it is time for your baby to twist and turn through the birth canal, flowing smoothly through, you let your body surge and push by itself. You let your mind rest deeply, trusting that the body know how to birth your baby, just as it has grown your baby moment to moment. Your mind rests as your body births your baby. Your body pulses naturally with the surges, giving your baby the perfect entrance into the world. *PAUSE.*

You bring your baby to you, skin to skin, your baby hearing your heartbeat and smelling you close by. You feed your baby to welcome him or her, and reassure your baby that you will still be nourishing your baby. You appreciate the work that your placenta has done in supporting and growing your baby. You give thanks to your amazing body. *PAUSE.*

As you get to know your baby, you know that you will soon know her or him better than anyone else. Your responsibility to this little being is strong and brings out your best qualities. You rest as much as you can, as you get to know each other, as you settle into feeding, settle into a new rhythm of life. In the birthing journey, you access parts of yourself that show you are strong, you have stamina, you are powerful. In caring for your new baby, you can be vulnerable and emotional. You ask for help when you need it. You take your time to adjust to being a mother (again). You honour your body, giving her time to be nourished, stabilise and strengthen. It took nine months to grow your baby and you give your body time to deeply recover. *PAUSE.*

Return to your intention about the pregnancy or birth. Think what your heart's desire is, in relation to the pregnancy or birth. You might repeat words, such as I trust my body to birth my baby, or remember a particular feeling or simply have an openness to your heart's guidance. *PAUSE.*

Have a sense of gratitude for having the wisdom to rest deeply and listen to this practice of Yoga Nidra in preparation for the birth of your baby.

Now return to the golden thread breath. Blowing out through soft lips. Let it carry you back as we come towards the end of the practice. Breathing a little more deeply, feel that as you breathe in, you draw energy, prana, into your body and to your baby. As you blow out the golden thread, or sigh, you are re-connecting with the world around you. *PAUSE.*

Become aware of your body lying in the room.

Now you feel ready to move, wriggling your fingers and toes, then moving your wrists and ankles.

You might like to rub your hand or hands around your beautiful belly. Keeping your eyes closed, you can hum on your exhalation, feel the vibrations moving down through your body, imagine your baby enjoying them. *REPEAT HUMS.*

Now, rub your hands together, producing some warmth and cover your eyes, gently massage the eyes. Then, slowly, slowly remove your hands letting in a little light, until you are fully back to the room, relaxed and refreshed. You may wish to eat or drink something to ensure you are reading for the rest of the day.

The practice of Yoga Nidra has now finished. Carry the benefits of the practice into the rest of the day or for a good night's sleep.